THOUGHT CATALOG BOOKS

More Than This

More Than This

KIM QUINDLEN

Thought Catalog Books

Brooklyn, NY

Contents

1

On Finally Coming To The Realization That Anxiety And Crohn's Are Intertwined

Kim Quindlen

I was diagnosed with Crohn's Disease when I was fifteen years old. I still remember sitting in a small room with cheesy cartoon wallpaper at my GI doctor's office, my parents sitting on either side of me, while my doctor told us in a solemn, steady voice that the results of my colonoscopy confirmed that I did, in fact, have Crohn's Disease. It wasn't exactly a scary or foreign concept to any of us. My mom's brother had been diagnosed when he was a child, and my cousin on my dad's side, who was my age, had been battling it since she was seven. So while the familiarity of the disease made things easier to understand, the actual diagnosis was harder to process (more so for my parents than for me), because they knew exactly what it was going to entail.

For me, it had been nearly a year of severe stomach pains, weight loss, complete and utter exhaustion, zero appetite, and—worst of all for a high school student—a horrible pattern of urgent bathroom trips. So as a naive fifteen-year-old, the diagnosis came as a complete relief. I thought *this is it, this is the problem! Now we can fix it!* First step was figuring out the illness, second step was swallowing a pill once a day, and then boom—life would go back to being totally normal. It helped that my mom couldn't keep herself from babying me during this period. She was constantly trying to feed me, encouraging me to sleep in as late as possible, occasionally buying me a new pair of jeans that she thought would cheer me up.

But eventually, after multiple trials of steroids and medications that didn't eradicate the problem, I realized that this wasn't going to be an easy fix. This was going to be more complicated than I thought. But still, I went through the first few years of my diagnosis with innocent eyes and a carefree attitude. Yes, when I was going through a flare-up, everything sucked. But I was still at a young enough age where I barely had any responsibilities, so when shit did hit the fan (pun kind of intended) everybody took care of everything for me. My dad could come take me out of school, my mom would call my doctor and sort out what we needed to do next, my teachers told me to take all the time I needed, and then I'd be sick for a couple days and allowed to sleep it off while everyone cooked for me and cheered me up. Young me always thought it would be this easy, until they inevitably came up with a cure in the next five years, of course! I don't think I ever consciously had that thought, but somewhere in the back of my brain, I remember comforting myself by allowing this belief to just float around and assert itself anytime I got worried.

College worked relatively the same way. It was a much

harder transition than I expected at first—leaving the doctor who had been our guide on what to do for the last three years, being 500 miles from home, unintentionally transitioning to the unhealthy diet of every college student, sharing a bathroom with twenty other girls. But I loved college so much that I got used to it, I got used to always feeling slightly awful and extremely lethargic. I was able to keep Crohn's relatively under control, or at least enough so that it didn't interfere extensively with my day-to-day living. So I ate and drank and partied like my body was invincible.

It was during my first couple years out of college that everything changed. The poor eating caught up to me. The lack of sleep caught up to me. The occasionally-forgetting-to-take-my-medicine caught up to me. The heavy drinking caught up to me. And, worst of all, the anxiety caught up to me.

I was twenty-three and preparing to leave my life in Cincinnati (I had moved there after college) to start a new life in Chicago, where I would chase after my totally unique dream of doing improv at Second City's training center. I had planned to go home to Atlanta for about a month in-between this transition. Instead, my body went haywire, and I ended up staying for four and a half months, forcing my parents to let me finally leave even though my body was still a complete mess.

It was like my body's normal way of half-functioning around Crohn's took it to the nth degree. Suddenly, I couldn't eat anything without severe stomach pains, nausea, or simply having the food go right through me. I would lay in bed for hours, only getting up when I needed to run to the bathroom (which was often every ten to fifteen minutes.) I couldn't keep weight on no matter what I did. I went on a diet that consisted of about ten things, and I hated it. I was irritable, depressed, panicked. I constantly felt like I couldn't catch my breath. And it was during this time that slowly, painfully, the anxiety of this disease began to trickle into my existence. No medications were working. The diet was as clean as possible and that wasn't working. Sleep wasn't working. The comforts of my family weren't working. I was beginning to grasp the fact that I was now an adult, that soon I would be in another new city by myself, that I was the one who had to figure things out now, and that the pleasant, floaty, comforting "they'll find a cure soon, this isn't a big deal" feeling was fully extinguished.

This was my life. This disease wasn't going anywhere. I had Crohn's, and I could no longer pretend that I didn't.

For weeks, even months, the anxiety ate away at me. When the flare-ups were particularly bad, when I was in so much pain that I could barely stand it, all I could think was *How can I possibly deal with this for the rest of my life? I could barely handle this day. How am I supposed to handle this for years to come? When I get married? When I have my own family to take care of? When I (hopefully) have a busy career? When I have to travel? When I'm invited on trips? How will I ever live a normal life when I'm too scared to even leave the house for fear of my body rejecting anything that comes into it?*

I kept these feelings to myself for a while. I was embarrassed, ashamed. I hated that I looked weak. I hated that I couldn't take care of myself, that I needed people. I hated that this anxiety had spread out comfortably at the center of my brain, that I could no longer remember how to breathe normally, how to think normally, how to leave the house without worrying about whether my body would cooperate. Why was I panicked all the time? Why couldn't I just get it together? My body was already out of control, why couldn't I at least control my mind?

Eventually, people who cared about me convinced me to start talking about it. To talk about all the frustrating and scary parts of this disease, to talk about how I was scared for the future, to talk about how much this disease made me need control and routine and consistency. How I was in pain. How it was normal that I felt panicked and uneasy much of the time. They talked me in circles, helping me to understand that the anxiety wasn't a different problem, another thing that I was doing wrong. It was part of this disease, it was completely wrapped up within it. It was normal to be anxious, it made sense to be anxious, I would be weird if I wasn't dealing with anxiety when it came to a disease where you felt like your body's behavior was unpredictable and all over the place. My parents, my boyfriend, my aunts, my siblings, my friends. Even a counselor that I begrudgingly went to for a couple sessions. They assured me over and over that this was just how it is. That this was my thing, the thing that I had to fight through. That I had to stop ignoring the anxiety and white-knuckling it. That I had to come to terms with the fact that it was a symptom of Crohn's, that millions of people deal with it in all sorts of ways, and that my way was that it manifested itself within the physical issues of my body.

I am still not healed. This is not an essay about triumph. I deal with the anxiety related to having Crohn's Disease every single day. I get panicked. I obsess over upcoming situations, particularly plane rides and vacations and small spaces and being in other people's homes. I worry about how my stomach will be in those situations. I have anxiety attacks in the middle of flare-ups. On particularly bad days when my stomach has a mind of its own, I have to occasionally take a Xanax just to handle the mental stress of being sick. I go to therapy sessions when things get dark.

But what I do have is this: awareness, knowledge, control over how I handle the lack of control. Even in the worst moments, when my body goes haywire and my mind is washed over with dread and anxiety, I know why it's happening. I know where the panic is coming from and I know when it will probably go away. I realize what it is, I understand the way that it works, I know how to cope with it. I know the safe foods to eat and the medicine to take and the shows that will make me laugh and the people that will cheer me up. It is not a triumph over the mental anguish, no. But it is an acknowledgement that I can stay afloat when the fear is trying to drown me. And although it's still a process, although some days I forget how to handle any of it, I'm still going, still moving forward, still leaving the house, still booking trips. Still a person outside of my body. Still a person outside of Crohn's.

2

The Fight For Control Of Your Own Body

Kim Quindlen

It comes in waves, at least for me. The anxiety, the worry, the obsession for control over my surroundings. The dozens of 'what if' situations that race through my head when I'm anywhere other than my home—particularly if I'm traveling, or staying at someone else's place, or at a crowded social event. *What if I get sick? What if I need to leave—where's my closest escape route? What if people think I'm weird for racing out? What if people notice I've ran to the restroom four times? What if I can't get in touch with my doctor while I'm on vacation? What if I have a really bad reaction to whatever meal I eat? What if people think I'm weird for barely eating anything?* I could write an entire essay alone listing all the what-if situations that run through my head on a daily basis.

But I've finally come to realize what I've needed to realize for a very long time: that the anxiety and the worries and the obsessions are not something that I will ever get over, or forget about, or defeat. Rather, they'll ebb and flow, just like the flare-ups themselves. It's the nature of the disease. Plenty of treatments, no cure. Good days, interspersed with bad days. Calm, lovely periods of health, followed by rushes of inflammation that come out of nowhere. It's always unpredictable, often random, always uncontrollable. The medications can help. The treatments and the surgeries and the procedures can help. Sometimes, you can even find something that works more wonders on your body and makes you feel better than you have in years (lookin' at you Remicade, champion of the GI tract). But nothing is permanent. Nothing is a guarantee. It's just a way to make things easier, more bearable, and sometimes, even downright pleasant if your body is feeling generous—at least until the flare-up subsides and you enjoy the peace before another round comes around.

I miss the control. I'd love it more than anything—to remember what it feels like not to have all these bizarre, in-depth, extremely specific worries about situations that may or may not ever happen. To not get stressed out about little things, like going on a road trip, or having friends stay with me, or avoiding certain foods while at a party and not wanting to have to explain why. It would be nice, it would be really, really nice, to be relieved of all that.

But this is the reality: I have this condition and it's not going to go away anytime soon. So while it feels good once in a while to imagine a life in which I didn't have these complications, it doesn't make me feel better in the long run. Because that's just daydreaming, and it's not going to get me anywhere. What helps me is this: Doing something. Making a choice. Accepting that I don't have control and then getting over it, even though I hate it and I hate the discomfort. Everybody who deals with this illness is different—everyone has different intensities of the disease and the inflammation, everyone has different ways of coping, everyone has different treatments, everybody has a different outlook depending on what they've been through. But I will say that what has helped me, at least mentally, is paying attention to the way my mind has grown, and expanded, and changed, because of this disease—particularly since my health has gone downhill in the last three years.

Now, I really don't care for the term "everything happens for a reason." I don't care to find a reason for the disease. That makes me feel like a chess piece or a person who just has to sit back and let things happen to her while she waits for someone to inform her of the reason for the way her body behaves. What I do find comfort in, however, is giving the disease meaning—meaning and significance that I decide on, because it's my brain and my body. A meaning, decided on by me, that gives back some of the control I've lost. I do not find joy from the disease, I do not find any pure, happy aspects to it. But I do find that I think differently because of it. The fact that I look happy, healthy, and strong on the outside—no matter how awful I am feeling internally—has helped me to comprehend, in a way that nothing else has, that there is so much behind every person that I meet. So many parts of their life I don't know about, so many things they've suffered through that I will never know, so many ways that their life is harder than my own that I can never presume to understand. It has kept me from lashing out at store clerks, or airline employees, or people on the bus, or friends, or simply a random person in a social setting that has irritated me in one way or another. I don't know what they've been through, I don't know what they're going through right now, I don't even know if they're feeling healthy and okay right in this very moment. I know nothing.

I have also learned that working hard, and putting all my effort into my job, and giving it my all when it comes to pursuing my passions, makes me feel lighter and freer than laying in bed and wallowing ever will. And yes, on certain days, when my stomach is acting like a little terror, all I can do is lay down and throw on an episode of one of my favorite comedies and try to sleep until the pain subsides. But for the most part, when my body is capable, I've learned that channeling my frustration and anxiety and discomfort into my work and my performances and my comedy makes me feel like something will come out of this. The fuel that comes from my desire to control something is giving this all just a little more meaning.

I've learned that nothing is more important to me than my relationships. I've learned that applesauce and Imodium and sleeping and an extra dose of Remicade can do a lot. But that at the end of a really bad day, all I really want is to call my parents or have my siblings send me funny texts or lay on the couch with my friends or have my boyfriend make me laugh when I'm half-delirious from exhaustion. I've received handwritten cards from aunts and grandparents during rough times and encouraging voicemails and 'thinking of you' mementos and nothing has helped me feel less isolated and less like I'm fighting this disease alone. I've learned what is most important to me.

The physical control is never going to come. Maybe in brief, occasional spurts, but that's it. For the most part, this is a lifestyle. This is just a way that I will be living, and that you will be living. So find your meaning, and within that,

you'll find other versions of control that you never even knew
existed.

3

The Challenge Of Learning To Let Someone Take Care Of You When You Find Love

Kim Quindlen

I've gotten used to the coping aspect of this disease. I've had it for long enough (eleven years) that I understand my version of 'normal' or 'healthy' is very different from that of a lot of people. Yeah, when it's bad, it's really bad. It sucks. But when it's just an average Crohn's day—a day where your stomach doesn't feel great and maybe it hurt a lot when you woke up—but a day when you can still eventually leave the house and work and do whatever it is that you need to do, you just get used to it. You learn how to go to the office or attend someone's dinner party or run your errands with a stomach ache, or a few trips to the bathroom, or just an intense urge to sleep for twelve hours. You get over it and you function around it.

You do this for so long that eventually you just learn to stop asking for help unless you really, desperately need it. Unless you're in a serious amount of pain. Unless you have no other option.

I know that part of me doesn't ask for help, doesn't like people taking care of me, and doesn't want to let people know when I'm sick simply because I'm stubborn. Because I want to just deal with it and get over it and then go to sleep and then start another day. But another part of me doesn't ask for help because that makes it real, that makes it a big deal, that makes people worry, that reminds me that I have a problem and that people are concerned about me because I have a concerning issue with my body. I like keeping it to myself sometimes because then it feels like it doesn't get too heavily involved in my life—I don't have to talk about it and I don't have to answer how I'm feeling every twenty minutes and I don't have to feel my mom's or my friend's or my sibling's worried glances on me when they think I'm not looking.

But I'm in love now, very in love. I am with someone who's in it for the long haul. I am in it for the long haul. And that changes things.

In any relationship or dating situation or casual fling that I've been in before, I've never bothered going into much detail (or, sometimes, any at all) about my condition. In my last relationship, he knew I had Crohn's Disease, he knew that I had stomach issues, and he would always do a good job of cheering me up when I was having a bad day. But the most detail I would ever go into was "I had a bad Crohn's Day today" and that was it. I left it up to him to figure out the rest or just read between the lines. I never talked about the emotional impact of it all, of the anxiety, of my worries for the future, of my worries for the present. I didn't talk about how difficult it was on certain days to get up and go to work. Sometimes when things were rough or I was feeling particularly horrible, I would cry in front of him. I would ask him to make me laugh or take my mind off of it all. But I never explained much about the reasons for my meltdowns, I just said the same old thing: "bad Crohn's day."

As for the other more casual, "we're talking" types of relationships, most of them never even knew. When we were hanging out or getting dinner or going out, I would smile and laugh and try to act light in spite of the sharp, stabbing pain in my left side. I would come up with ridiculous, long-winded reasons as to why I had to suddenly leave the bar. I would cancel dates or plans if things were really bad, saying that I had the flu or something else that sounded a little more cute than "sorry, I'll be on the toilet all night!"

There's a strong sense of shame, for myself and for a lot of other fellow patients I've spoken with, about this illness. There's an embarrassment about the nature of the disease. There's a hesitation to talk about the symptoms. There's a desire to deal with it on your own. There's a dread of having to bring up your doctor's appointments or your specific and strict diet regimen or any particular needs/routines you need to have when it comes to things like traveling. We just don't want to do it, we don't want to have to involve others. And we especially don't want to have to deal with it when a significant other is involved. Who wants to say "I've pooped fourteen times today" when someone you are extremely attracted to asks you what's wrong?

But I've been with my boyfriend for three years now, and the moment I realized I wanted to be with him for life (which happened very quickly), was the moment I realized that Crohn's was going to play a part in the equation. I couldn't hide it, I couldn't play happy when I felt awful, I couldn't keep lying and making up excuses for why I didn't want to go places and do things. He knew from the start that I had Crohn's Disease. But telling a significant other you have this illness usually happens in two parts. First, you just tell them you have this condition and that it's a chronic inflammatory disease and blah blah blah. You make it sound as medical as possible. And then you tell them what you really have: you talk about the pain and the bathroom urgency and the digestion problems and the exhaustion and the joint pain and the mood swings and all the other unsexy things that happen with your body.

And then you have to learn to let them take care of you.

Sometimes that means letting them cook for you, pick up your safety foods at the grocery store, grab medicine from the pharmacy. Hand you a few blankets when you can't stop the chills, grab you a cold pack when you can't stop sweating. Marathon a show with you when you're too beat to do anything else. Fill up your cup for you so that you don't get dehydrated. But that's just the first level of letting someone take care of you.

The second part, and what I will argue has been even the more crucial part for me, is letting them take care of you when you feel like you're about to lose your mind. When you're anxious or beaten down or tired of feeling horrible and you just need someone to vent to, to talk to, sometimes to cry to. Someone you trust enough to have a meltdown with. Someone to talk you off the ledge when you're convinced you'll never get better. Someone to go with you to your infusions or doctor's visits or any other procedures you may have. Someone to protect you from the isolation that this illness tries to throw on us so consistently.

When things are really bad, yeah, you need someone to physically take care of you. To check your fever, to feed you, to grab you whatever you need. But for the most part, you're tough. You've learned how to deal with this. You can whip up some scrambled eggs and fill up your water bottle and sleep it all off until you get better.

But no one can replicate the comfort and reassurance you can find from a significant other when it comes to dealing with Crohn's. Their pep talks, the grip of their warm hand in yours, their company on bad days, their capability of reading your face in social situations and knowing when you need to go home, the things they do to make you laugh when it's the last thing you feel like doing. The feeling of being so close and so understood by another soul brings a kind of comfort that is stronger than any steroid a doctor can throw at you.

It takes a while. It takes trust. It takes a lot of embarrassing and uncomfortable conversations. Conversations that you'll soon learn (if you're with a good one) are no big deal at all to them, regardless to how ashamed and 'gross' you may feel that you're coming across as. But when you get passed it, when you tell them you have Crohn's Disease and then when you tell them you have Crohn's, what you're doing is giving yourself a better chance at a normal life, a better chance at happiness, one more way that you refuse to allow this disease to fully take over your life.

I still hate it sometimes. I still occasionally feel awkward and embarrassed when my boyfriend is over and I'm feeling quite under the weather. I tell him that I hate it and it's awkward and I don't want to talk about it. But then he tells me that he doesn't care that I'm being "poopmotional." And then I laugh at his joke and the sound feels wonderful coming out of me. And then I lay against his warm body and I feel that, at least in this moment, he is keeping the typical, crushing isolation of the illness at bay.

4

What You Should Know If You Fall In Love With Someone Who Has Crohn's Disease

Kim Quindlen

They're tough, because they're used to being scared and uncomfortable and in pain. But that can be tricky. They've learned how to fend for themselves, so sometimes, it might take them a little while to learn how to let you take care of them too.

They're fighters, they're survivors, because this disease doesn't have a cure. There's no specific path that works for everyone. There's no single answer. So they've learned how to figure this thing out for themselves—how to find the perfect balance in their treatment that allows them to live a life as close to normal as possible.

There were probably time periods in their life which they were very okay. Sometimes periods of wellness that even lasted for years. But there's also been times where their health has been taken away from them. They've learned to fight for it. They've learned to fight for health and happiness and whatever else will allow them to feel joy in their lives. Often, that includes love. They will fight for you, if you make them feel good and light and carefree and beautiful and joyful and healthy and all the other things that they don't feel in the dark moments where the flare-ups are uncontrollable and their stomachs hurt and they're afraid of food and they're afraid to leave the house.

Those dark moments really are quite dark sometimes. Painful and frustrating. Sometimes, they won't feel like fighters. They will feel weak or sad or angry or afraid of their own bodies. They will try to avoid pity parties and meltdowns, because they know deep down that that will only push them back further. But sometimes, they will not be able to help it, because they are weak and tired and human and they are angry about the bodies they've been given.

Sometimes there will be nothing you can do to help. You will see them in pain, and you will want to fix it. You will want to take it for them – to get rid of their abdominal cramps or their long days of upset stomachs or the sharp pain that jabs into their sides and wakes them in the middle of the night. But you can't. You will not be able to fix it. You cannot fix their bodies.

What you can do is hold them. Brush your fingers through their hair. Soothe their nerves. Remind them that they are not alone. Sometimes, the hardest part about this all is the isolation. The endless time in the bathroom. The desire to hide the illness from others. The anxiety and the shame. The frequent need to turn down trips or social outings or fun evenings at a restaurant, because their stomach can't handle it and all they can manage to do is lie in their bed for hours, trying to sleep through the pain and hoping that tomorrow will be better.

They feel so alone a lot from it all. That's often harder than the cramping and the urgency and the pain and the worry. It's the fact that they feel like their burden is invisible and nobody can understand it. Sometimes the most important thing you can do is to remind them that they are anything but alone.

There will be beautiful days, though, too. Days where they appreciate the sun and the warmth and the joy of being outside more than most people, because they are so happy to be up and about and feeling strong and alive. They love the sun, they love the beautiful days. But they don't need them to appreciate the beauty of life. They're not put off by rainy days or cold winds or dark clouds, because nothing's darker than having to waste the day in a bathroom or their bed or the hospital, wondering when they will be able to go out and experience the world again. The don't need a beautiful day to realize it's a beautiful day. And you will be the person they want to share it with.

They've already seen themselves in their darker moments, and they know how to appreciate the thrill of living. The thrill of experiencing the world. The thrill of falling in love with you.

They will love you fiercely. They will laugh with you always. They will appreciate you and be grateful for you, because they understand how precious happiness is.

They will love to love you. But there were also be ugly moments. They will go through a lot of ups and downs and there will be lots of fears and uncertainties. They will have other issues that sometimes come along with Crohn's. Like anxiety. Constant exhaustion. Depression. Arthritic pain. Issues with various foods. A weak immune system.

It's an ongoing disease, it's an ongoing fight. They're strong, but sometimes this disease sucks out so much strength that they will have moments of fragility in which they will need you more than you could ever imagine. They don't need you to heal them or fix them or take care of their problems.

They don't want you to pity them or feel bad for them or baby them or let them get away with things.

All they want is you, holding them in both the beautiful and the ugly moments, reminding them how wonderful it is to be alive and reminding them that they are not alone. Because when you're with them, it will help them to believe that tomorrow will be a beautiful day. That's all they need.

5

What You Should Know If Your Best Friend Has Crohn's Disease

Kim Quindlen

They're going to depend on you a lot, even more so than they let on. And it's not that you have to do anything more than just be a normal friend. The reason they love you is exactly that: you make them feel normal. You bring a sense of routine into their life.

You're consistent. You're dependable. You're something that they understand and you're something that makes sense, and that's something they can't count on in their own body. Their body is a lottery—anything could happen at any moment, and they really have no way of predicting it. So being around someone like you, someone who makes them feel safe and light and happy, is sometimes better than all the Remicade and Prednisone and Mercaptopurine and Humira in the world. (Although, these magical potions are definitely a plus.)

When you have a disease that, for the most part, is not life-threatening, you feel both incredibly blessed and incredibly lost in terms of what to do. For the most part, there is no short-term, all-consuming, stressful fight to survive, and for that, Crohn's patients are incredibly grateful.

But the hard part is coming to terms with the fact that, for the rest of your life, you will be fighting through unpredictable periods of ups and downs. Flare-ups. Never-ending medical trials, where you're trying not to get your hopes up but you're praying that—just maybe—this one will work, at least for now. You'll try diets and supplements. You'll have anxiety in all aspects of your life: work, social gatherings, airplanes, vacations, road trips.

Having Crohn's as a lifelong companion is an unfortunate realization that every patient has to acknowledge. Because, at least for now, there is no cure. Crohn's is just something that each patient is learning how to work into their life. Something that they're doing their best to adapt to and to be proactive about, because the last thing they want to do is to spend their life in a vacuum of self-pity.

And that's where you come in. You bring in a bright light, a feeling of normalcy, a much-needed sense of calmness when they're on the verge of hyperventilating or having a meltdown or simply feeling like they're not a match for their own frustration.

They love you for understanding, for being discreet when they need to leave a party or go home early from work or skip out on an event altogether. The fact that they don't have to explain anything to you is a godsend, and they'll appreciate it, and you, more than you'll ever know.

Whether or not you realize it, you're being one of the most incredible friends in the world, just by being there. Just by providing them with a sense of continuity and regularity. Just by making them laugh and reminding them that, although you'll never be able to fully relate, you understand that they need you and you know how to remind them that they aren't alone.

Your normalcy is a gift. Your loyalty is a gift. Your simple presence has the power to put them at ease. You're a gem. And you're very much appreciated for it.

6

Going To College With Crohn's Disease

Samantha Fudge

For most people, college is scary. It's overwhelming, it's a whole new chapter in their life. It's hard to move away from your parents, your friends and your hometown. It's terrifying to venture out by yourself and learn how to live on your own. From living with a family to having your own responsibilities of cleaning, cooking, laundry and much more, it is a big change. But for most people, college also brings with it excitement. It is a place to start over. A new life with new people. A place to reinvent yourself and to discover new passions. College was both of these things for me. But then you add in a disease that I still don't have under control or completely understand (and I don't know if I ever will), and that just adds in a whole new layer of anxiety about college. Moving to college and adjusting to it was tough, but getting my Crohn's to adjust was even tougher.

Freshman year I moved into my dorm at Simmons College. I'm from Everett, MA, so moving to Boston didn't seem like such a big deal. I felt excited and couldn't believe that I was old enough to be living on my own. I knew I would miss my family and my friends, but college had advertised so many differ-

27

ent possibilities that I couldn't wait to get started. I ended up hating freshmen year. I made friends and I loved my roommate. My classes were interesting, and I even joined some clubs. But I hated it. The switch from high school at home to college was no joke: the workload increased like crazy, the dorm life never offered any privacy, and doing things like laundry were harder than I expected. I would get sick a lot because of the stress, and I couldn't figure out a way to explain to my friends what exactly was wrong.

Crohn's is often associated with a gross stigma because it is a stomach disease, and hey, shit doesn't smell like roses. I found myself sugarcoating my symptoms, saying that Crohn's just made me tired a lot and that I would occasionally get stomachaches, hiding the fact that five minutes after every meal I would end up sick in the bathroom. Embarrassed to the point that I would run downstairs from the third floor every half hour to use the private restroom. I couldn't do things that my friends could. I didn't have the energy to go out and party every weekend; I couldn't sip on the horrible beers we were served at frat parties without having to throw up. I hid these symptoms, trying so hard to blend in and be normal, and becoming miserable in the process. I ran home a lot, to my family who understood what my disease was. I hated college.

Then, the second semester of freshmen year, my friends and I decided to head to Southie for the St. Patrick's day parade. We stayed out all day, partying and goofing off, living the life of a Boston college student. The next morning, I woke up throwing up blood. Scared as hell, I called my mom and she rushed me to the doctors. I was admitted for about a week, and the GI team performed many tests. I was having a Crohn's disease flare-up. That week in the hospital was completely miserable, but it opened up a door for me. I realized I couldn't really hide my disease anymore, that it was a part of who I am. As much as I hated its symptoms, they couldn't be ignored or sugarcoated. Crohn's disease is serious, and I realized that the hard way. It was time to come clean and explain the extent to which this disease ran my life. I opened up, and I explained how Crohn's affects me, and I finally became more comfortable with it.

Now, almost two years later, I am beginning my junior year of college. I am a proud advocate of Crohn's Disease and have raised a lot of funds through programs such as Take Steps and Team Challenge. All of my friends know about my disease, and they respect it. I'm not embarrassed anymore to say "Hey guys, my stomach's killing me, I'm going to stay in tonight," or "Hold on guys, I need to run to the bathroom, Bartol dinner went right through me."

I'm not uncomfortable to talk to my professors, to let them know that I will need to leave class often to use the bathroom, and that some days I won't even be able to pull myself out of bed for class. Of course it still sucks that I am more restricted than my friends and that I never seem to be able to do everything they can. But, it's getting better. Crohn's has forced me to grow up quickly, and to become my own advocate. As I am writing this, I have been in bed all day because I was up all night throwing up. But unfortunately I can't sleep anymore. College keeps moving no matter what disease you have, and I have a huge load of homework to get done. Crohn's is part of me, and I have fought to get it under control and to be able to do all of the fun college things that I want to. I have a great group of friends here, and I have my family at home. I lucked out with two amazing support networks.

7

A Reminder That Crohn's Is Something You Have, Not Something You Are

Kim Quindlen

You are not Crohn's Disease. You are not an illness or a statistic. You are not a success story or a sob story. You are not a weakness or an embarrassment or a disability. You are not a joke. You are not a body that sits in a hospital room, waiting for a doctor to come in, to look you over without really seeing you, to assign one more medication to you.

You are a person. You are a person who has a chronic illness. You, yourself, are not an illness.

It can be hard not to become the disease, especially when you've spent countless hours having to explain to friends and coworkers and bosses and significant others why you can't come into work today or why you can't go out tonight or why you can't make it to their birthday celebration.

When a significant portion of your life is focused around Remicade infusions or Humira injections or a Prednisone trial or just finding something that will work—even just for now, so that you can leave the house—it can be hard not to completely associate yourself with the disease. It can be difficult not to base your entire identity around this illness.

You want Crohn's Disease to just be another something about you, like your hair color or your height or your age. You want it to be a careless fact—I'm blonde, I'm 5' 3", I have Crohn's Disease. But it can be hard to tack it on as *just another thing about me,* when you're spending such a significant amount of your time worrying about getting sick in social situations and finding food that doesn't make you ill and stressing out about traveling and scheduling multiple doctor visits into your busy weeks.

Sometimes, there are steady periods where you can forget about it for a little while. Not completely, but at least to the point where you can go out without needing an escape plan, where you aren't thinking about Crohn's the minute you wake up. These are beautiful, brief oases that give you time to think about the disease, to process it. You wonder how you could have ever been that caught up in the illness, you question if maybe you were just being a little bit dramatic.

And then the flare-up comes back, as it always will, and it's really all you can think about. Your days revolve around food, or a lack of desire for it, and sleeping, and bathroom breaks, and excuses. Fake reasons about why you have to leave work or the party or the event early. Sleepless nights and wanting-to-sleep-all-day days.

These are the moments where it is so easy to become the disease. It takes up such a large space in your mind, because of the worrying and the planning and the anxiety. Often, by accident, this illness becomes the only thing from which you derive your sense of self.

When I feel this starting to happen to me, I try to remember what what my doctor told me 9 years ago, right after I was diagnosed: "You have Crohn's Disease. Crohn's Disease does not have you." A cheesy statement, maybe. But real nonetheless.

Crohn's often takes away your control. So you try to get that control back by finding a sense of identity within the disease. *I was diagnosed this many years ago. This is how I deal with it on a daily basis. This is what I eat. These are my medications. These are the issues I have. These are my side effects.*

Crohn's tries to trick you. Crohn's tries to make you think that this is who you are. But what you need to remember is that you exist outside of this illness. You can find your sense of identity from who you are and what you do *in spite of* having Crohn's Disease.

This is not to say you should walk around like a martyr, patting yourself on the back and informing everyone of what a warrior you are. Yes, your suffering is real, and at times it has probably been very intense. But everyone has issues, everybody has a cross to carry.

Crohn's is one of your crosses, one of your challenges, one of your issues. It will probably be a steady companion throughout your entire life. Sometimes it will be in the background, sometimes it will be right in your face, refusing to be ignored.

Don't try to avoid it. Do everything in your power to make it easier on yourself. Do everything in your power to take care of your body. Don't try to hide the pain, just acknowledge that it's part of your reality and keep going.

Refusing to allow Crohn's Disease to become your identity doesn't mean you have to ignore it. It is a significant part of your life, and you can form a safety net for yourself when you need it—discovering safe foods that you can eat, putting on your favorite show when you need comfort, getting extra rest when your body is exhausted, turning to people you can count on when you need to be encouraged.

The illness is real and it always will be. The medications are real, the side effects are real, the exhaustion is real, the flare-ups are real. But they are just the things that make up your cross. They are not you.

You are the person who's living and creating and experiencing and doing and trying, in spite of the fact that Crohn's is trying to pull you back. Some days you will feel weak. Some days you will feel strong. Some days you will feel mediocre, just somewhere in the middle. That's okay.

What matters is just that you keep going, that you keep living, that you keep doing things that will help remind you that you exist outside of this box.

You have an age. You have a height. You have an eye color. You have Crohn's. These are all just things about you. Perhaps Crohn's affects you more than some of your other characteristics, but it is not you. It never will be. And as long as you can remember that, it will never beat you.

8

Uplifting Mantras To Remember On The Days When You're Feeling Particularly Awful

Kim Quindlen

A combination of my own oft-repeated mantras—that I've either made up myself or subconsciously retained through the advice and comforting words of others over the years—as well as some of my favorite quotes from some of the world's best thinkers on how to handle your body and your mind on your worst days.

1. You have survived plenty of days like this before, and you will get through this one, too. It may not be pleasant, it very well may be painful and uncomfortable. But your mind is stronger than you realize, from having gone through this so many times before. You can do this.

2. Remember to breathe. Always remember to breathe.

3. You are not alone in your suffering. There are 1.4 million people in the United States alone dealing with IBD and everything that comes with it. Take comfort in the fact that other people have what you have, that other people struggle too, that there are others in the world who know exactly what you are dealing with, and that you are not weird or weak for sometimes feeling upset and discouraged.

4. This illness is bringing you more knowledge, more wisdom, and most of all, more compassion that you realize.

5. People love to say that laughter is the best medicine. Personally, I'd feel better with a solid dose of Prednisone or Remicade or Humira. But the unexpected rush of a bubble of laughter in my throat can make me smile even on the worst of days. It's what I like to think about when things are particularly dark—memories of laughing until I cried with someone who makes me smile.

6. This is not who I am, and it never will be. It does not define me. And still, I am stronger because of it.

7. "Bad times have a scientific value. These are occasions a good learner would not miss." —*Ralph Waldo Emerson*

8. There are a hell of a lot of things that seem a whole lot less scary now, because I've been through this and I continue to get through it every day.

9. This, too, shall pass; this, too, shall pass.

10. You will learn more about yourself and who you are in these awful, difficult moments than you ever will in moments that are easy, blissful, and happy. You will discover new perspectives and new ways of thinking because you are suffering. And although any of us would choose optimal health if we could, we can't. But at least we can search for new knowledge and understanding while we are struggling—and come to realizations that we never would have come to otherwise.

11. "Being challenged in life is inevitable, being defeated is optional." —*Roger Crawford*

12. Tomorrow might be hard too. But there's also a big chance that it will be a better day. And it's okay to focus on that if it will get you through today.

13. "With the new day comes new strength and new thoughts." —*Eleanor Roosevelt*

14. Everybody has hard days, weak days, horrible days, I-don't-know-if-I-can-do-this days. And sometimes what you need to do is swallow your pride and swallow your stubbornness (at least, I'm speaking personally here) and reach out for comfort from someone who makes you happy.

15. "If you aren't in over your head, how do you know how tall you are?" —*T.S. Eliot*

16. Our bodies are not permanent. Our minds will last far beyond this. At least, that is what I believe, and that's what gets me through a lot of the darkest moments.

17. You are always, always stronger than you think.

18. "Let us rise up and be thankful, for if we didn't learn a lot today, at least we learned a little, and if we didn't learn a little, at least we didn't get sick, and if we got sick, at least we didn't die; so let us all be thankful." [*Sometimes I love this quote. But to be fair, sometimes I hate it.*] —*Buddha*

19. "So far you've survived 100% of your worst days. You're doing great." [*An anonymous and popular phrase that I think of often, and which, out of everything, brings me the most amount of comfort.*]

9

Thank You For Loving Me In The Ugly Moments (A Love Letter To My Person)

Kim Quindlen

I wish I wasn't sick. I think about it pretty much every day—what it would be like to feel wonderful and healthy and strong all of the time. To never be tired. To not be afraid of food and how my body will handle it. To not feel scared every time there's a sharp pain around my stomach. But surprisingly, I know you wish this for me even more than I do. I know, without a doubt, that more than anything, you wish you could take it from me. You look at me in my hardest moments, and you don't have to say it, but I know what you're thinking: you would do anything to take it on yourself and leave me painless.

It could be so much worse. It's not debilitating (for the most part). It will not kill me. I will get through it and I will live a very normal life. But there are very ugly moments, moments that most people don't see. It's an invisible illness. I look healthy on the outside. So the ugly moments go unseen by pretty much everyone but you. The difficult moments build up one on top of another, to the point that every few months, it gets to be too much and I break down in front of you and no one else. I cry and I'm angry and I become child-ish—I get frustrated that I have to deal with this and I feel bad for myself and I tell you that it's all too much to handle. When I get upset like this, it's the most pained I've ever seen you look.

Yesterday we sat in a room that smelled like antiseptics and Clorox wipes. You smiled and made jokes with me and made me feel like I was a normal person who just happened to be in a slightly abnormal situation. We laughed in the middle of a hospital room, while a nurse hooked me up to an IV. She apologized while she jabbed a needle in my arm, but I barely paid attention. I was too busy laughing at you, as you tried to be supportive while simultaneously trying not to faint from looking at the needle. You gave up your Saturday, no ques-tions asked. You've done it before and you'll do it again. You woke me up with a full breakfast, because you didn't want me to be hungry during this long day. The monthly visits to get my infusion medication have become routine, but I still dis-like them. You know they scare me a little bit, but that I'm too proud to admit it. So you grab my hand the minute we sit down, and you act like you're doing it absentmindedly. But I know you're doing it so that I won't be scared.

The infusion is tiring. My arm is sore. They pump me with Benadryl too, so I'm in and out of sleep the entire day. But every time I wake up, you're there. Sitting next to me in your cheap, uncomfortable chair. Reading a book, lost in your own world. But smiling reassuringly to me each time I open my eyes. Answering the nurse's questions for me when she comes over to get my vitals. Speaking in that low, calming, knowledgeable tone of voice that you have. I doze the entire time we're at the hospital, always feeling a comforting sense of peace, because I know you're right next to me.

I'm not a good enough of a person to say that I'm actually, truly "thankful" to have Crohn's disease. But what I can say is that I'm aware of the realizations it's brought me to. It's reminded me of how lucky I am to have you in my life. Most people could only ever dream of being with someone like you. You're not romantic in the most common sense of the word, but my definition of "romantic" has changed since I've been sick. You've made the 30-minute drive to my apartment at midnight when I've had a particularly straining day. You've learned everything you need to know about my diet, so you can cook meals that I can actually eat without feeling sick. You know how to comfort me when I have really bad days, without allowing me to fall into the easy trap of pitying myself.

It's a tough disease. It's ugly and scary and it can get in the way of trying to feel normal. But it has shown me what a special person you are. How lucky I am to have you. What's actually important in a relationship. The type of person I should want to be with.

You don't just love me when we're in the hospital room or when I'm laying in my bed, where the setting is strangely tender because I'm weak and hopeless and you know that I need you. You also love me in the moments that aren't romantic. Like when I've gone through several tough days or weeks, and I've been cranky and angry and a nightmare to deal with. And I've taken it out on you, because you've loved me enough to stay there with me while I've been at my weakest point.

This isn't a phase. It's a lifelong illness. Sometimes I will be okay. But sometimes, I really won't be. And you know that. And you've seen the times when I'm really not okay. And you stayed. You comforted me and you loved me even when I was being a brat. You've taken care of me, but you've also refused to allow me to feel bad for myself. You've forced me to acknowledge that I have an illness without letting the illness have me. You've loved me in the ugly moments. And that's my favorite thing about you.

10

Sick Of Being Sick (Or, How I Learned To Stop Worrying And Love My Bowels)

Eliot Rose Dreiband

When I sat down to write this essay I had this funny image in my head: I am standing at a podium in a nondescript school auditorium facing three rows of blurred faces seated in folding chairs. All very Alcoholics Anonymous-esque.

"Hi, I'm Eliot and I have Crohn's Disease," I say to the faces. "Hi, Eliot," echoes back at me.

"I was diagnosed with Crohn's Disease when I was 12 years old. It is an incurable, autoimmune disease that affects your gastrointestinal tract...I was diagnosed with Fibromyalgia at age nineteen. Fibromyalgia is a disorder characterized by widespread muscle pain and fatigue. I have..."

I am almost monotone in my description of my incurable genetic illness. It's come to the point now where I'm almost sick of talking about Crohn's Disease. This clingy, needy, temper tantrum-ridden Gollum has attached itself to my body for over half of my life now and I'm a little sick of it. But I have to

talk about it. Crohn's Disease is something I deal with contin-
uously and it's clawed its way into all aspects of my life.

From the basics: my saying "no" to those delicious-looking
chili cheese fries. ("Your recipe has beans? Can't. Thanks any-
ways!") To the routine: scheduling treatments, doctor's
appointments, and prescription refills like an octogenarian.
Only you're 25 and have no idea how health insurance actually
works. To the embarrassing: Going home sick from work
because you can't stop feeling nauseous (for no known reason)
and you don't want to throw up in front a client (this almost
happened...twice).

Now add Crohn's to dealing with insurance companies, job
decisions, traveling plans, relationships, etc. Oh and add two
other diseases, because these auto-immune illnesses tend to
be systemic. See? It goes on and on. You'd get sick of talking
about it too. But I have had this illness now for over half my
life, it is second nature and has influenced too much of me.

One of the reasons I'm sick of talking about my illness
is because it's really important to me not to complain about
too much about myself. Everybody's got something. So by all
means complain a little. But no one person can claim all the
world's suffering and there are a hell of a lot of people who
have things worse off than me. I try to save my breath for
more interesting conversations than my illnesses.

But I also like to think that I'm that getting sick of talking
about my diseases because I no longer define myself by them.
I was diagnosed with Crohn's Disease as a pre-teen, a veritable
identity-molding age. I had blood tests, doctors, and insurance companies telling me that I was unhealthy and abnormal
and then I had to turn around and relay that information to

my friends and teachers to explain my absences and symptoms. Needless to say, it led to a lot of conflicted feelings about my identity, my weaknesses, and my strengths. And oh boy, do I have the teenage, angsty journal entries to prove it.

I have spent a lot of time and energy making sure that people do not view me as vulnerable because of my illness. At 5'3" I am already aware of my stature limitations, but I don't like the idea of that people assume less of me because of the cards I was dealt. What might be intended as sympathy can come off as pity.

But therein lies the rub. Having a disease does make things in life harder. It can be painful, exhausting, frustrating, and embarrassing. A disease is a stressor both to the inflicted and those around her. I hate that I have been such a financial burden to my parents, though they would not think twice about it. And I can't even count the number of times I've had to cancel or postpone plans with friends because of sudden symptoms. A good excuse or not, my disease's negative repercussions don't make me feel stronger as an individual.

So what does make me feel positive about my illness? I like to think it had a pretty big effect on how I choose to live my life and interact with people. Rebecca Chapman and I first at a camp for children with Crohn's Disease and Ulcerative Colitis. We were 13, newly diagnosed, and terrified. But being around other children with these illnesses alleviated my anxieties and let me just relax, have fun, and be a kid. I returned every summer to the Painted Turtle Camp until I was old enough to volunteer—and I still volunteer with them to this day. The Painted Turtle Camp's mentality and values alongside my experience dealing with an illness have made me a more empathetic and socially motivated person. In college I changed my major to Human Development and Human Rights and in the future I'd like to work in the social justice sector. I'm even leaving in a few weeks to go volunteer in Buenos Aires, Argentina for three months with a children's rights organization.

I guess that's when you know that you have wonderful friends and family—when they can joke about your incurable illness without making you feel like less of a person. The Gollum-esque creature I like to think of as my negative symptoms is my friend's interpretation of my disease. She talks about Crohn's Disease with absurdly anthropomorphic phrasing. According to her my "immune system hates me and therefore has declared a mutiny" on my bowels. My brother has mentions my "pill popping habits" loudly when I pull out my medications with breakfast in public. Having an illness can get a little too serious. I'm glad I have people to help me bring a little levity and laughter to the matter.

Nelson Mandela said that, "It all seems impossible until it is done." Now, I'm almost 100% positive that Nelson Mandela didn't have Crohn's Disease, but lucky for me his message still applies. Having Crohn's Disease and Fibromyalgia is a pain, quite literally. But I try to give myself a break while still moving forward. Having wonderful people in my life who inspire and love me keeps me positive, happy, and healthy. They not only remind me to take my pills and avoid popcorn, but that I am human and allowed to be a little vulnerable.

11

But The Fighter Still Remains

Jessi Moss Glasscock

I am 32 years old and the mother of five children: boy/girl twins that are eight, my youngest girl that is six, and two step-daughters ages fifteen and nineteen.

And I also have Crohn's Disease.

I had my first two babies in 2007 but had suffered from the awful symptoms of Crohn's since my first few years in college. Miraculously, my body was able to carry twins full term and I had a healthy pregnancy and delivery. I also carried my third child full term, but my pregnancy wasn't as easy as it was with the twins. I stayed sick throughout the nine months and had a horrible time trying to gain weight for the pregnancy because of constant trips to the bathroom. It wasn't until after my third child that I got my diagnosis in February of 2010. Finally, I knew what I was up against and would be able to start fighting this disease head-on.

Over the years I've been on many different regimens. I've been on Humira, Remicade, Cimzia, multiple rounds of Prednisone, Flagyl, Cipro, Methotrexate, Bentyl, gluten free and organic foods only, and currently the only medication I'm on is Entyvio. I've been on this infusion med for over a year now, and for a while it worked great. But over the Christmas season of 2015, I noticed a lump of some sort in my lower abdomen area. I had an MRI a few weeks ago and the results weren't great. That lump is a loop of bowel that is coming through the muscle lining of my abdomen. There is new disease showing on the MRI and scar tissue that's beginning a formation of a blockage. I have a colonoscopy that is scheduled in two days so, of course, the anxiety is setting in. First off, anyone that's had a colonoscopy knows what the day before is like—pure agony. And with being a mom that works out of the home and has children that are involved in extracurricular activities after school, the thought of a colonoscopy prep makes my heart race.

My kids have grown up watching me struggle in my day to day life and having to miss out on many activities because I just couldn't leave the house or not be in close proximity to a toilet. I can only imagine what their thoughts consist of when they think of Crohn's Disease. Dealing with this disease can be full of stress, full of anxiety, and full of humiliation at times, but all of these negatives make you appreciate the good days even more.

Before Crohn's Disease I was pretty carefree. I went with the flow and really wasn't a "planner." Now, after dealing with this disease for so long, I kind of have to plan. You have to know your limits. You have to know where every bathroom is within a fifty-mile radius. You have to learn when to say "no." You have to realize that on any given day, everything that you had "planned to do" may have to be cancelled due to a flare-up. But you also have to be open and honest with people. I know some people choose to deal with their disease on their own and keep it to themselves. But I have learned over the years that it's best to just get it out there in the open. With myself, I always have so many comments made about my weight. I'm almost 6' tall and I weigh about 125 pounds. When people meet me they usually ask, "What's your secret to staying so skinny?!" and my response is usually pretty blunt: "Crohn's Disease." Sometimes people know exactly what the disease entails. Others have no idea and you have to go through the explanation of the disease. At first, yes, I was very uncomfortable telling people about all of the symptoms that I deal with on a regular basis. But after the first few times it got easier, and now it's just like regular conversation.

Crohn's Disease is a part of me, but it's not what defines me. Yes, some days are pure hell. I sit up in the bed at my 6 AM wake-up alarm and wonder how on earth I am supposed to get through this day. Those days you sometimes feel defeated, but it's how you respond to those hellacious days that truly shows you what you're capable of. I, for one, am not going to let this disease stop me from enjoying life. You have to commit yourself to surviving minute by minute, hour by hour, and then day by day. You learn exactly what you're made of, and to be honest, anyone with a chronic condition that can "fake it 'til they make it" is an all-star in my book.

Many days you have to get up, dress up, and show up, and sometimes that's all you can do—the necessaries of your day-to-day life. Other days you will wake up feeling like you can move mountains. On those days, I push myself—sometimes more than I should, but those good days are appreciated so much more because I know what defeat feels like.

My kids deserve to have a mom that will show them what

determination looks like. They deserve to be able to do all the extracurricular activities that all the other kids do, even though it's a struggle most days and the chronic fatigue takes me over at times. It is my responsibility to show them that you can accomplish anything you set your mind to despite the circumstances of your life. They need to know what it looks like to never ever give up hope. If you give up, then they will give up too. Crohn's Disease can teach your kids compassion, motivation, determination, empathy, and many other qualities that most parents want their kids to possess. If there is one thing that I want my kids to learn from my disease, it is to NEVER, EVER lose hope. There will be brighter days ahead when you're walking through the storms and valleys. You will overcome your biggest fears if you never lose sight of hope. Your strength will prevail and the fighter inside of you will always remain.

12

Face Your Fears Head-On, And You'll Have Nothing Left To Fear

Erin Ann McCarthy

Though it didn't start out that way, my life in New York City turned into a constant struggle. A struggle to make ends meet, a struggle to ever relax, a struggle to attain personal fulfillment.

When I was 23, there was no place more exciting, no place filled with more possibility than the Big Apple. I felt motivated and driven to keep up with the pace of it all. It became a place in which I learned to assert myself and to gain independence. After a couple of years, however, I found it an ever increasingly difficult place to live, day in and day out. To call it "home" was a struggle. The fading of the honeymoon period became palpable. Instead of looking forward to Friday night amongst the glittering lights and 2am subway rides, I just wanted to hide. Daily life became exhausting. From the moment I stepped out of my cramped living space to greet the day, I dove head first into a current of competition. From the crowded sidewalk to the crowded subway, I entered survival mode adorned with my "armor." Stone face, headphones in. I was impermeable. Or so I thought.

I didn't realize at the time that I was battling through life instead of enjoying it. I have no doubt that a small part of me knew it wasn't the right way for me to live, but I chose to ignore it. Mostly because I thought that I was doing what I was "supposed to do." And if I gave up, I would be perceived as weak. New York is supposed to be the place where you make a name for yourself, where the world is your oyster. Life is hard, and New York just seemed to make it that much harder for me. It took spending a week in the hospital for me to realize my life needed to change.

In the winter of 2013 I became severely ill. I was diagnosed with Crohn's Disease and spent a week in the hospital. I was unable to take care of myself, plain and simple. It was humbling to watch my body fail me. I had a difficult time understanding why I could become so paralyzed by illness after everything I knew about living a healthy lifestyle. But nonetheless, I needed help. I couldn't do it by myself. My body was screaming out in pain for me to listen to it, to make a change. I don't use the word epiphany flippantly, but I had one when I was in the hospital. I vowed right then and there that I was going to live my life for me. In that moment, I no longer felt scared or paralyzed by fear to make a decision about my future. It was time for a big change. Up until that point I had seemingly made choices that were wrong for my innate personality and for my life's desires. Instead of focusing on who I was, I was consumed with "what" I was. I had ignored what kind of life would make me happy. And my body was telling me: enough.

I believe we prevent ourselves from making big life changes because the routine structure of life makes us feel safe and secure. But that is a complete illusion. What is more difficult is to make choices that will benefit you, even if they seem frightening at the time. I decided to buy a one-way ticket to San Diego, and I've never looked back. What I was seeking was a more balanced and healthy lifestyle. To get that, I needed to get out of New York.

To be sure, I still have moments of frustration when dealing with my chronic illness. Moments of denial. But it remains a part of who I am, and I don't let it define me. I try to live with it instead of against it. We all have our crosses to bear, and I happen to wear mine on the inside. The nature of my condition presents a life that is unpredictable, which is why I try to live my life in the present. The illusion of permanence exists for everyone. We don't really know where life will take us, so it is essential to focus on what is happening right now. Today, I am healthy. I don't know what tomorrow will bring but I can't let that ruin what I have today.

In times of great difficulty, there is always light amidst the darkness. With pain, there is love. These dualities are what life present in order to encourage us to shift our perspective. We can relieve ourselves from suffering by refusing to resist what is and make choices that enrich our soul. For me, it was to move across the country in order to make myself a priority. Live your life authentically, and doors will open up opportunities that you could have never imagined.

13

On Becoming Vulnerable In Love

Jessica Plummer

When I was first coming to terms with my Crohn's-Colitis diagnosis, one of my greatest fears was being unlovable. I thought that I was way too much to handle. I could barely take care of myself; why in the world would someone emotionally invest in me when most of my focus was just trying to get through the day or take care of my responsibilities? It was during my college years when things were the worst, the times of "Ring by Spring" at my college, where you couldn't escape the pressure of marriage. I was watching people get engaged at a ridiculously rapid rate and the idea of dating wasn't even an option for me. I was too busy being hospitalized every other week. I was barely passing my classes and writing term papers heavily medicated and somewhat high on morphine.

I struggled with depression and found myself self-medicating. I wasn't taking my prescription painkillers to alleviate the pain; I was taking them because they made me feel emotionally numb. I stopped taking them cold turkey when I realized what I was doing, and of course the pain continued to be excruciating. Sometimes, I wouldn't change clothes, much less shower on a regular basis, because I wanted to scream from the arthritis and intestinal pain I was experiencing.

I was never particularly confident growing up, but before the hospital visits in college, I was a serial monogamist. I always had some sort of guy in my life. It was new for me to feel completely unwanted or unloved. I was everyone's sick friend. I was one of the guys. I was used to being the tomboy, but it was very lonely not to have any sort of indication that I was still worthy of love or a relationship with a significant other or that anyone was even the slightest bit attracted to me. But who would be attracted to their sick greasy friend who's secretly covering up her odor with deodorant and perfume?

After two years, I became comfortable with the idea of not being in a relationship. I was focusing on my career and getting through school. It didn't occur to me that being in a relationship was still on the table. It also didn't occur to me it would be way more challenging than not being in one.

I met my boyfriend Wyatt on an internet site that no longer exists. I refer to it as eHarmony's bastard child—jazzed.com. I created an account out of loneliness. Most of my free time I spent just existing because I didn't have the energy to do much outside of school, work, and internships. I longed for companionship, even if it was superficial internet conversations. Sure, I had friends, but I learned quickly that friendships in adulthood took way more effort to maintain than in adolescence. Not everyone wanted to lounge around with the sick girl on their weekends off (but I cherish the friends who did.)

But one unexpected day, I received a message from this goofy guy writing about the lack of character development of Snuffleupagus in *Sesame Street* Season Six. We would message back and forth and I found myself laughing out loud at the silly things he would say. I didn't know that almost six years later, we would be living together with our dog Tyga.

We could not be more opposite. He is a gym rat, a personal trainer, and his background is in health and nutrition. I was the sick girl who ate whatever it was she was allowed to despite whether or not it was nutritious. Going to the gym would just make me sleepy and I would want to nap on the equipment. When we first started dating, we lived an hour away from each other and we only saw each other on weekends. Our limited communication and lack of quality time complicated us really getting to know one another. I was impatient with him and his lack of understanding of myself or my illness. He was impatient with me when I didn't fit the guidelines of a typically-healthy human being. We fought about my eating habits. He struggled to understand my various symptoms. He would get mad at me if I didn't want to eat because he didn't understand that sometimes eating would only make my nausea worse. He once said to me, "If you don't want people to think you are anorexic than you should eat something." That was one of the most hurtful and ignorant things someone has ever said to me since my diagnosis.

I wanted him to be a mind reader. I wanted him to just know when I wasn't feeling well. I wanted him to understand all of my non-verbal cues. I didn't want to have to tell him what I was feeling and when. I pretty much wanted him to be psychic. It took a long time for me face this unrealistic reality and I recognized I needed to start communicating what I was feeling. Communication has never been my strength. Especially when you have a chronic illness that is gross and uncomfortable and goes against societal norms of what's "okay" to talk about.

We have come a very long way since then. He started googling my illness and taking the time to understand what it all meant. He started taking mental notes of what foods I could or couldn't eat. I started communicating my symptoms. We had a few hiccups along the way—like when he would tell me what I was or wasn't "allowed" eat, but I would eat trigger foods anyway because I knew the risk and didn't care if I was going to get a stomach ache afterwards. We struggled going out to eat with his friends or family. It was hard enough for me to be vulnerable with him, much less having to constantly be the center of attention and asked the "So, what CAN you eat?" question. I hate this question. I loathe this question. But, I have learned it is a necessary evil. He continues to lecture me because I struggle/don't bother to prep meals for myself when I get into situations where there may not be food available for me to eat.

One of the unexpected challenges I continue to struggle with is that my boyfriend and I should be in our prime with young thriving sex drives. Well, he has quite the healthy sex drive. Me, not so much. My chronic fatigue overpowers any sort of sexual desire I might have. For a while, he perceived this as being a manifestation of my lack of sexual attraction to him. He doesn't understand 100% what it is like for me, but at least he now understands that my fatigue is so overpowering, it is difficult for me to want to engage in sexual activity. This continues to be an area I struggle with, but I have found that talking about it at least helps. After attending my best friend's

Pure Romance party, I have learned there are products out there to help assist with this type of stuff, so I am still hopeful.

But despite all the challenges, one of the greatest things that has come from my relationship is realizing and accepting that I am more than my illness and that I am enough. Does having a chronic illness complicate things? Absolutely. I struggle when I am too tired to spend quality time together or cancel plans. I sometimes put overwhelming pressure on myself to be entertaining and energetic all the time when my body is desperately trying to shut down. But with some feedback from my therapist—"you are not a cruise director on a ship, relationships are a two way street"—I am learning it is not my job to be energetic and happy all the time. It is my job to be me and it is my job to be vulnerable enough to let my significant other see my whole self, including my weaknesses.

My bond with Wyatt is deeply rooted in our desire to be silly and childlike with one another. We joke around constantly, particularly about my illness. It has been the greatest coping skill I could ask for. I created the Hashtag #cuteselfieonthetoilet to help normalize bathroom talk. I post my colonoscopy pictures on social media. I talk about my yogurt poop, or my rainbow-colored poop, and describe my intestinal pain in the most graphic detail to help others understand what I am going through—i.e. describing my intestinal pain as my intestines being shredded by a blender and ripped out of my body. I have stopped caring if my reality makes others uncomfortable and it's been the greatest thing for me.

Once I stopped letting my disease be an excuse for a wall between my boyfriend and me, our relationship flourished. It is now just a normal part of life and doesn't interfere with how we engage with one another. He is there for me when I need support giving myself injections. He cooks me dinner or runs errands for me when I can't get myself out of bed. He constantly reminds me that I am worthy and I am so much more than my illness. He loves me even when I don't shower for a week because I'm having a flare. If that's not love, I don't know what is.

14

Here's Why Crohn's Disease Can Be Beautiful If You Want It To Be

Kim Quindlen

Crohn's Disease is not something you win against or something you beat. You can go into remission at times. You can make it through a flare-up to the other side. You can have phases where you only have to see your doctor every few months instead of every couple of weeks. But Crohn's is always there, hanging over you like an oppressive cloud. A cloud that you completely dread, but one that feels uncomfortably familiar at the same time.

That unsettling familiarity comes from the fact that Crohn's is with you at all times, no matter how hard you work to control it. You can have the cleanest diet in the world and the strongest medicine possible for your body (Remicade or Prednisone or Humira or an infinite number of others), but Crohn's doesn't ever fully go away. You can keep it at bay. You can feel better than you have in years. But it's still always right there, ready to pounce at any moment.

It's especially noticeable in the big moments, even if you feel that you're at your healthiest. The minute you plan a vacation, or get on a plane, or are offered a new job, it slinks into the room as a dark shadow that cannot be ignored. You're imagining every possible circumstance, wondering what you could possibly do if your body decides to act up. And the answer is usually: nothing.

And even in the not-so-big moments, when you're trying to relax on a Saturday or are just showing up at work for another 'ordinary' day, it can show up. And it's isolating and exhausting and nerve-wracking. You're out of the moment—just counting down the hours until you can go home and lay in your bed, or spending your Saturday evening wracking your brain for what you could have possibly eaten that destroyed your stomach today.

But as loud as Crohn's is to you, it's a fairly quiet disease to everyone else. The symptoms aren't stereotypically visible, besides – possibly—fatigue. Even if you have scars, or a bag, from a surgery, they're mostly hidden, seen only by the people closest to you. That makes your situation hard to explain, hard to relate to, and hard to translate to a person who has a clean bill of health.

So when these things happen (mostly regularly), it's tempting to let Crohn's turn you into someone ugly. It's frustrating when doctors ask you to rate your health on a scale of 1 to 10, because you can't really remember what 'normal' is supposed to feel like; your 'normal' is not everyone else's normal. So it feels good to get angry, and to feel bad for yourself. It's easy to let yourself sleep all day every day. It's just simpler to give in to your situation and let it become who you are, rather than looking at it as just one aspect of you.

But even if you don't believe that everything happens for a

reason, even if you don't believe in God or any sort of higher being, you can still take power from your situation. You can look at the way it's affected your life and the perspective that it's given you, and refuse to let it be something that's only impacted you in a negative way.

Would you change it if you could? Of course you would. You would get rid of this thing faster than you can say 'colon.' But because you can't (at least for now—come on, Science!), you can find power in other ways. The ability to control your body is out of the question, but what you can do is learn to appreciate the mindset you've developed from having a chronic illness.

Sure, you're tired a lot. And angry, and worried, and jealous of those whose bodies can do what yours can't. But you're also probably tough. You've been in a lot of pain before and you've gotten through it. You've learned that if you want something, you have to be the one to make it happen, because there will be a million things trying to prevent you from getting it.

You appreciate your good health when you have it. You can see most days as beautiful even when they're rainy or stormy or freezing, because feeling well enough to leave the house is all you need for a day to be considered lovely.

You probably find it easier to relate to others who are suffering—even if their version of suffering has nothing to do with what you yourself have been through. You have probably found a deeper sense of empathy, because nothing helped you more in your darker days than someone who made you feel less alone—even if they didn't understand in detail what you were going through.

You don't have to believe that you have this illness because it was 'meant to be.' You don't have to believe that it happened for a reason—that it was the will of God or the universe or any other being. Regardless of your spiritual beliefs or lack thereof, you have the power in this situation—not to cure yourself, but to give your illness meaning. To take advantage of the perspective that healthy people don't have. To appreciate the lens through which you look at the world—the one that causes you to be more tough and determined and curious and kind and awake.

When I was debating trying Remicade, a friend with Crohn's said, "It helps a lot. You'll look around and think 'this is how normal people feel all of the time!'" He was right in one sense. After a few infusions, I was feeling better than I had in awhile; I felt almost as good as a normal person (though the effects have lessened since I started).

But here's the thing. I don't think anyone is actually 'normal.' We all have unique perspectives because we've all been through something or a lot of things. We've all suffered in one way or another. We're all strong in different ways. It's whether or not you choose to finding meaning within your suffering that sets you apart.

Crohn's is your thing. Crohn's is your outlook. And you can let it control you, or you can make damn sure that the pain you feel only makes your world more lovely.

About the Author

Kim is a writer and comedian living in Chicago. She grad-
uated from Miami University (no, the one in Ohio) in 2012
with a degree in English/Creative Writing. After graduating,
Kim decided to try stand-up comedy. Being a middle child,
she naturally fell in love with the attention. She's continued to
explore her interest in comedy which has led to performing
improv around the city of Chicago and writing full-time for
Thought Catalog. She spends her free time trying to befriend
cats at house parties.

Thought Catalog, it's a website.

Social

Corporate

www.ingramcontent.com/pod-product-compliance
Lightning Source LLC
Chambersburg PA
CBHW050512290526

45786CB00007B/2530